www.facebook.com/offici

CANCER CANCER CANCER:

Curing Cancer Using Cannabis -

The Wondrous Healing Properties Of Essential Oils and Tinctures, The Rick Simpson Story, And Other Cries Of Miraculous Healing!

By King Cajun

www.crushitwithkdp.com

◆◆◆

Copyright © 2015

www.crushitwithkdp.com

www.facebook.com/officialbookpageforcuringcancer

TABLE OF CONTENTS

DISCLAIMER:

COPYRIGHT:

NOTE FROM THE PUBLISHER:

INTRODUCTION ABSTRACT

CHAPTER ONE: BRIEF HISTORY AND CONTROVERSY

CHAPTER TWO: CURRENT USES FOR CANNABIS AS A MEDICAL TREATMENT

CHAPTER THREE: MEDICAL RESEARCH FOR CANNABIS AS A TREATMENT

CHAPTER FOUR: PRESENT DAY OPINION AND USE IN THE UNITED STATES

CHAPTER FIVE: THREE CASE STUDIES FROM AMERICAN SURVIVORS

APPENDIX:

RESOURCES: FIND YOUR SENATOR HERE!

REFERENCES:

www.crushitwithkdp.com

www.facebook.com/officialbookpageforcuringcancer

Disclaimer:
Although the author and publisher have made every effort to ensure that the information in this book was correct at press time, the author and publisher do not assume and hereby disclaim any liability to any party for any loss, damage, or disruption caused by errors, editorials, or omissions, whether such errors, editorials, or omissions result from negligence, accident, or any other cause.

NOTE FROM THE PUBLISHER:

Join us on our mailing list either on Facebook or our website. As a thanks from us for signing up you can download your free copy of "25 Tasty Treats For Your Holiday Table"

So go here and sign up!
http://www.crushitwithkdp.com/thankyou

This will automatically register you for FREE GIVEAWAYS in the future! EVERYONE IS A WINNER!!! You will be entered to win as soon as you sign up on our Facebook fan page OR SIGNUP at our website - so sign up, subscribe, LIKE, comment, SHARE, SHARE, SHARE, and stay tuned for more details!!!

Email us at kingcajun@crushitwithkdp.com We try to respond within 3 days but sometimes it takes a little longer.

http://www.facebook.com/officialbookpageforcuringcancer

DubC Haynes, Editor

www.crushitwithkdp.com

www.facebook.com/officialbookpageforcuringcancer

KingCajun Publishing

Thank You for Your Support!

Y'all come back now, ya hear?

http://www.crushitwithkdp.com

http://www.kdpmoneymachine.com

www.crushitwithkdp.com

www.facebook.com/officialbookpageforcuringcancer

<u>Copyright © 2015 by TBHCLLC</u>

All rights reserved. This book or any portion thereof may not be reproduced or used in any manner whatsoever without the express written permission of the publisher except for the use of brief quotations in a book review or scholarly journal.

First Printing: 2015

ISBN-13: 978-1514349502

ISBN-10: 1514349507

KingCajun Publishing

123 William Harris Road

West Monroe, LA 71292

www.crushitwithkdp.com

www.kdpmoneymachine.com

skype: xxbadbillyxx

www.crushitwithkdp.com

www.facebook.com/officialbookpageforcuringcancer

Before we get into the meat of the book on curing cancer we wanted to let you know that you can start eating the Paleo Way and gain many health benefits very easily. Your body will benefit from the natural way you will learn to eat.

Today we wanted to share with you a little gem we've found that has helped many people on a number of occasions. We would not share or endorse this if we didn't believe you would greatly benefit from this information.

It's called The Paleo Grubs Book, and it's hands down the number one resource we use on a daily basis to not only make Paleo work, but to make it work more easily.

Some key features of the book:

Over 470 Recipes – Sure, there are plenty of recipes online for free, but when you want consistent results, you have to trust your source. Detailed pictures and simple steps make all the difference.

Desserts are Included – We wouldn't have lasted a week on Paleo without a steady stream of waistline friendly desserts. Don't use willpower; satisfy your cravings for the sweet stuff.

Crock Pot Recipes Make Paleo Easy – Includes a separate recipe guide full of slow cooker Paleo dishes that puts your success on autopilot. Spend less time cooking and still lose weight and look great.

Hate following recipe instructions? It's probably not your fault, but the recipe itself. The instructions in this book are easy to follow, so much so that even we were surprised.

www.crushitwithkdp.com

www.facebook.com/officialbookpageforcuringcancer

And the photos are professionally taken, so they'll spur you on to create what you see.

In case you haven't noticed yet, The Paleo Grubs Book gets our highest recommendation or it would not be in this book and if you want to try it out you get it instantly, so you can cook up your first recipe tonight while you're still excited.

One thing we've found, this book has actually saved us a lot of money, not only in the form of time, but also because:

– You won't waste money buying unneeded items at the grocery store.

– You'll learn how to make your own food from scratch rather than buying pre-packaged items.

– You'll save yourself from the head trip of having to plan out your meals every day or week.

It's basically a lifestyle upgrade that takes the Paleo diet from being a confusing and stressful monkey on your back to a simple and easy-to-follow plan that you can use to create the body you've always wanted.

Click here to download the Paleo Grubs Book
http://bit.ly/kingcajun

Any affiliate links in this book go to help support our efforts in spreading the good news. Please click through and visit the offer as we truly believe you will benefit from it and It will help us continue to publish quality content.

www.crushitwithkdp.com

Introduction Abstract:

The following e-book argues for the use of Cannabis as a treatment option for Cancer and other diseases of the body. While Cannabis treatment remains controversial and the United States and in places across the globe, medical research continues to explore and support use in many cases. This eBook will focus on several cases of successful use of Cannabis in the United States in alleviating and treating disease and will provide a description of the current atmosphere in the United States. Recent research and commentary from physicians and organizations supporting use and an appendix of resources will also be provided.

Chapter One: Brief History and Controversy

On August 7th 2013, a news article on CNN opened America's eyes to the journey of Charlotte Figi, a young 6 year old girl who has Dravet Syndrome, a rare form of epilepsy. The Figi's treatment options took a turn, after being inspired by the story of Jayden David, reported by CNN in December of 2012, another child with Dravet Syndrome, whose father reported successful treatment of his son's seizures with medical marijuana since June, 2011. The Figi's, after trying "every other option" began working with two physicians licensed in Colorado to provide medical marijuana to their daughter (Sanjay, 2013). Charlotte's parents reported, at the age of five, she was having 300 grand mal seizures a week and was in hospice preparing for an order her parents placed, "do not resuscitate" (Young, 2013). After working with the physicians and a growing operation and dispensary in Colorado, the Figis found a variety, which now carries the name of their daughter, which reduced Charlotte's seizures to two per three a month (Young, 2013).

While the use of Cannabis as a treatment option for diseases such as epilepsy and Cancer remains controversial in the United States (and countries across the world), medical research and survivor reports continue to explore and support the use of Cannabis in many cases. Nearly half of U.S. states allow marijuana to be used medically and testimonials from Cancer survivors are ubiquitous on the Internet. Controversy around the use of Cannabis stems mainly from the United States decision to effectively criminalize and restrict possession of and heavily tax authorized medical and industrial uses with the Marijuana Tax Act of 1937 (Frontline, 1998). Upon enactment of federal laws, by the mid-1950's a first-offense marijuana possession in the United States carried a minimum sentence of 2-10 years with a fine of up to $20,000 (Frontline, 1998). Up until the Tax Act of 1937, "marijuana was one of the top three medicines prescribed in the U.S." (Genetic Science Learning Center, 2014). Much of the present day controversy around medical marijuana stems from fear of the drug being more readily available as a recreational drug as a result of increasing its use medically. Fears around recreational drug use include: lingering beliefs around marijuana as a gateway drug, concerns about use by youth (including concerns around cognitive development) and the likelihood that some people unknowingly use marijuana to mask, or self-medicate, for physical and mental health problems, including depression, anxiety and insomnia.

    The first case since the Marijuana Tax Act of 1937 began restricting marijuana use in the United States to reverse the tide was the of Robert Randall, a Washington, DC man who suffered from glaucoma. When Judge Washington dismissed criminal charges against Randall, he became the first American to receive marijuana treatment for a medical disorder (www.druglibrary.org, 2010). Throughout the 1960's and early 1970's efforts to criminalize marijuana possession and use waned, but in 1984, under President Reagan and the Anti-Drug Abuse Act, mandatory sentences for drug-related crimes were enacted. The Act implemented the same penalty for 100 marijuana plants and 100 grams of heroin and provided the death penalty for "drug kingpins" (Frontline, 1998).

President Reagan signed the Anti-Drug Abuse Act, instituting mandatory sentences for drug-related crimes. In conjunction with the Comprehensive Crime Control Act of 1984, the new law raised federal penalties for marijuana possession and dealing, basing the penalties on the amount of the drug involved. Possession of 100 marijuana plants received the same penalty as possession of 100 grams of heroin. A later amendment to the Anti-Drug Abuse Act established a "three strikes and you're out" policy, requiring life sentences for repeat drug offenders, and providing for the death penalty for "drug kingpins" (Frontline, 1998). In 1996, Proposition 215 was passed in California allowing for the sale and medical use of marijuana for patients with AIDS, cancer, and other serious and painful diseases. Currently, the law stands in tension with federal laws prohibiting possession of marijuana (http://vote96.sos.ca.gov/bp/215.htm).

Part of the tide against marijuana, also began in 1970 when the Controlled Substance Act was enacted. This act labeled cannabis as a drug with a high potential for abuse and "no accepted medical use" (Genetic Science Learning Center, 2014). The potential for abuse and the labeling of the drug as a gateway drug have been chief arguments against legalization of medical marijuana, with little differentiation in past legislation between medical and recreational use. The majority of the arguments against the medical use of marijuana stem from the implications of marijuana use as a recreational drug. In fact, as of April, 2015, federal Judge Kimberly Mueller declined "an order to remove marijuana from Drug Enforcement Administration's list of most harmful and addictive drugs" (http://topics.nytimes.com, 2015).

In a statement on the Office of National Drug Control Policy for the U.S. (www.whitehouse.gov/ondcp, 2015), the opinion of the Federal Government is made clear:

> "The Administration steadfastly opposes legalization of marijuana and other drugs because legalization would increase the availability and use of illicit drugs, and pose significant health and safety risks to all Americans, particularly young people."

In the public eye of opponents and in the opinion of the U.S. Federal Government, legalizing marijuana for medical use will "increase availability and acceptability" will lead to higher public health costs, will increase dependence and addiction, particularly among the young and will create an increase in health issues and a decrease in cognitive functioning (Whitehouse, 2015).

While it is recognized that the use of marijuana for medical treatment is controversial, this eBook will argue it is viable treatment for disease of the body, including epilepsy and Cancer. Additionally, the e-book will provide a brief history, an explanation of the current uses and purposes, a description of the present-day US atmosphere, three case studies of Cancer survivors and a final appendix of resources.

Chapter Two: Current Uses for Cannabis as Medical Treatment

Google "current uses for Cannabis as a medical treatment" and you will return about 61,800,000 results in 0.56 seconds (Google.com, accessed May 7, 2015). Increasingly, respected organizations and physicians throughout the U.S. are citing (and some emphasizing) the use of medical marijuana to treat disease. According to the American Cancer Society (American Cancer Society, 2015), Cannabis can treat a host of symptoms in regards to patients with Cancer, including, but not limited to:

Treating nausea and vomiting from chemotherapy
Treating pain caused by damaged nerves
Improving food intake
Requiring less pain medication

Additionally, the American Cancer Society cite research that THC and other cannabinoids such as "CBD slow growth and/or cause death in certain types of cancer cells growing in laboratory dishes" and that "some animal studies also suggest certain cannabinoids may slow growth and reduce spread of some forms of cancer" (American Cancer Society, 2015). Other disease symptoms that can be eased from marijuana cited by the American Cancer Society include improvement of appetite for HIV patients, treatment of seizures, reduction of inflammation in the body and serve as an antioxidant.

In 2004, Former US Surgeon General Joycelyn Elders, MD, made similar claims in an editorial published by Providence Journal:

"The evidence is overwhelming that marijuana can relieve certain types of pain, nausea, vomiting and other symptoms caused by such illnesses as multiple sclerosis, cancer and AIDS -- or by the harsh drugs sometimes used to treat them. And it can do so with remarkable safety. Indeed, marijuana is less toxic than many of the drugs that physicians prescribe every day."

In a Huffington Post article, Andrew Weil, MD (2010) noted that in addition to known uses of medical marijuana today, that an American doctor of the late 1800's would use Cannabis for treating symptoms of everything from labor pains to nervous disorders. On Dr. Weil's website, he states the Cannabis can also be used to treat sleep disorders, epileptic seizures and multiple sclerosis and is one of the lower rated substances for risk of addiction (http://www.drweil.com, accessed May 7, 2015).

The National Cancer Institute cites numerous clinical trials and meta-analyses that "have shown that dronabinol and nabilone are effective in the treatment of N/V induced by chemotherapy" (www.cancer.org, accessed May 7, 2015). Dronabinol is a synthetically produced delta-9-THC. THC or tetrahydrocannabinol is the chemical responsible for most of marijuana's psychological effects and belongs to a class of compounds called cannabinoids. In addition to its psychological effects, the compound also has a multitude of medical uses. THC was approved in the United States in 1986 as an antiemetic to be used in cancer chemotherapy. Made available in Canada in 1982, Nabilone, a synthetic derivative of delta-9-THC is now also available in the United States (www.cancer.org, accessed May 7, 2015).

Pain management is also a focus of work presented by The National Cancer Institute (NCI). Improves a patient's quality of life throughout all stages of cancer. Cancer pain is known to result from inflammation in bones, nerves and other pain sensitive areas. Severe and persistent pain it is often resistant to treatment with opioids. Citing the results of three studies (two of which were double-blind placebo-controlled), NCI reported that "15 mg and 20 mg doses of the cannabinoid delta-9-THC were associated with substantial analgesic effects, with antiemetic effects and appetite stimulation" (www.cancer.org, page 5, accessed May 7, 2015). In the third, follow-up single-dose study, it was reported that 10 mg doses of delta-9-THC produced analgesic effects during a 7-hour observation period that were comparable to 60 mg doses of codeine, and 20 mg doses of delta-9-THC induced effects equivalent to 120 mg doses of codeine (www.cancer.org, page 5, accessed May 7, 2015).

In an editorial in the *Boston Globe* titled "Marijuana as a Wonder Drug" (2007) Lester Grinspoon, MD, of Harvard Medical School, wrote:

"The mountain of accumulated anecdotal evidence that pointed the way to the present [marijuana as treatment for HIV neuropathic pain] and other clinical studies also strongly suggests there are a number of other devastating disorders and symptoms for which marijuana has been used for centuries; they deserve the same kind of careful, methodologically sound research.

While few such studies have so far been completed, all have lent weight to what medicine already knew but had largely forgotten or ignored: Marijuana is effective at relieving nausea and vomiting, spasticity, appetite loss, certain types of pain, and other debilitating symptoms. And it is extraordinarily safe -- safer than most medicines prescribed every day. If marijuana were a new discovery rather than a well-known substance carrying cultural and political baggage, it would be hailed as a wonder drug."

In a recent report, it was reported that due to "medical science is strongly in favor of THC laden hemp oil as a primary cancer therapy", not just in a supportive role to control the side effects of chemotherapy, that The International Medical Verities Association "is putting hemp oil on its cancer protocol" (Sircus, 2014). Before its popularity as a recreational drug, the hemp plant was used in elixirs and medicinal teas because of its healing properties. According to Sircus's cite, hemp oil can be used in many nutritional and trans-dermal applications.
Rick Simpson, a cancer survivor well-known for his efforts to educate the public on medical marijuana primarily by sharing his own journey, makes his own hemp oil for oral

intake and claims in small doses it does not have the psychotropic effects, yet works for healing disease. On his website, phoenixtears.ca, Simpson provides information on using hemp oil for a variety of disease, including, but not limited to:
- treating and controlling cancer
- reducing pain
- relief for arthritis
- treatment of asthma
- antibiotic for infections
- lowering blood pressure
- treating depression
- treating insomnia

Additionally, Simpson includes information on how to produce the oil for medical use on his site, at http://phoenixtears.ca/make-the-medicine. Essentially, to make the oil, Simpson claims one must follow these steps (as summarized by Walia, 2014) at:

To make Rick Simpson's hash oil, start with one ounce of dried herb. One ounce will typically produce 3-4 grams of oil, although the amount of oil produced per ounce will vary strain to strain. A pound of dried material will yield about two ounces or roughly 60 grams of high quality oil.

IMPORTANT: These instructions are directly summarized from Rick Simpson's website. Be VERY careful when boiling solvent off [solvent-free option], the flames are extremely flammable. AVOID smoking, sparks, stove-tops and red hot heating elements. Set up a fan to blow fumes away from the pot, and set up in a well-ventilated area for whole process.

1. Place the completely dry material in a plastic bucket.

2. Dampen the material with the solvent you are using. Many solvents can be used [solvent-free option]. You can use pure naphtha, ether, butane, 99% isopropyl alcohol, or even water. Two gallons of solvent is required to extract the THC from one pound, and 500 ml is enough for an ounce.

3. Crush the plant material using a stick of clean, untreated wood or any other similar device. Although the material will be damp, it will still be relatively easy to crush up because it is so dry.

4. Continue to crush the material with the stick, while adding solvent until the plant material is completely covered and soaked. Remain stirring the mixture for about three minutes. As you do this, the THC is dissolved off the material into the solvent.

5. Pour the solvent oil mixture off the plant material into another bucket. At this point you have stripped the material of about 80% of its THC.

6. Second wash: again add solvent to the mixture and work for another three minutes to extract the remaining THC.

7. Pour this solvent oil mix into the bucket containing the first mix that was previously poured out.

8. Discard the twice washed plant material.

9. Pour the solvent oil mixture through a coffee filter into a clean container.

10. Boil the solvent off: a rice cooker will boil the solvent off nicely, and will hold over a half gallon of solvent mixture. CAUTION: avoid stove-tops, red hot elements, sparks, cigarettes and open flames as the fumes are extremely flammable.

11. Add solvent to rice cooker until it is about ¾ full and turn on HIGH heat. Make sure you are in a well-ventilated area and set up a fan to carry the solvent fumes away. Continue to add mixture to cooker as solvent evaporates until you have added it all to the cooker.

12. As the level in the rice cooker decreases for the last time, add a few drops of water (about 10 drops of water for a pound of dry material). This will help to release the solvent residue, and protect the oil from too much heat.

13. When there is about one inch of solvent-water mixture in the rice cooker, put on your oven mitts and pick the unit up and swirl the contents until the solvent has finished boiling off.

14. When the solvent has been boiled off, turn the cooker to LOW heat. At no point should the oil ever reach over 290° F or 140° C.

15. Keep your oven mitts on and remove the pot containing the oil from the rice cooker. Gently pour the oil into a stainless steel container

16. Place the stainless steel container in a dehydrator, or put it on a gentle heating device such as a coffee warmer. It may take a few hours but the water and volatile terpenes

will be evaporated from the oil. When there is no longer any surface activity on the oil, it is ready for use.

17. Suck the oil up in a plastic syringe, or in any other container you see fit. A syringe will make the oil easy to dispense. When the oil cools completely it will have the consistency of thick grease.

For even further information, check out Rick's written recipe here.

On this page of his site, Simpson includes dosage information http://phoenixtears.ca/dosage-information/ which is an important component of using marijuana to treat disease.

Chapter Three: Medical Research for Cannabis as Treatment

Research supporting the use of marijuana medically is widely-available. While there is scientific work available on a variety of disease, the following chapter will focus on Cancer, providing a background for the patient stories presented in chapter five of this e-book. One of the most valuable resources accessed in the writing of this eBook is the website www.procon.org, established in 2004. While a host of other sites and books exist, and are provided in the resources section, this chapter will focus on the peer-reviewed studies from 1990 to present, as presented by procon. Of the seven cases reviewed by procon.org involving cancer (as treatment or for symptoms), five of the studies found the use of medical marijuana could benefit cancer patients, as either a potential treatment, or more often than not, as a drug to help treat symptoms. While fewer studies report the benefits and recommend use, most of the studies recognize the proliferation of anecdotal evidence and most argue that with such limited scientific research, the benefits are outweighed by the unknowns of the use of medical marijuana for treatment of epileptic seizures at this time. Three of the seven studies clearly suggest marijuana "may have a place in treatment" (procon.org, 2015).

Study Name*	Type of Study	Finding Results
Pathways Mediating the Effects of Cannabidiol on the Reduction of Breast Cancer Cell Proliferation, Invasion, and Metastasis	Peer-Reviewed, Pre-Clinical	General consensus in the field of cancer research is "that targeting multiple pathways that control tumor progression is the best strategy for the eradication of aggressive cancers. Since CBD (Cannabidiol) has a low toxicity, it would be an ideal candidate for use in combination treatments with additional drugs already used in the clinic. Importantly, CBD appears to be interacting through a cellular system that regulates the expression of key transcriptional factors (e.g., Id-1) that control breast cancer cell proliferation, migration, and invasion. The experiments described in this manuscript not only define the pathways that CBD is working through to control breast cancer cell aggressiveness, but also demonstrate the efficacy of CBD in pre-clinical models. A greater understanding of this system may lead to future therapies for breast cancer patients, including the additional refinement of CBD analog

		synthesis."
Preliminary Efficacy and Safety of an Oromucosal Standardized Cannabis Extract in Chemotherapy-Induced Nausea and Vomiting	Peer-Reviewed, Clinical, Double-Blind	"Despite progress in anti-emetic treatment, many patients still suffer from chemotherapy-induced nausea and vomiting (CINV). This "pilot, randomized, double-blind, placebo-controlled phase II clinical trial designed to evaluate the tolerability, preliminary efficacy, and pharmacokinetics of an acute dose titration of a whole-plant cannabis-based medicine (CBM) containing delta-9-tetrahydrocannabinol and cannabidiol, taken in conjunction with standard therapies in the control of CINV."
Multicenter, Double-Blind, Randomized, Placebo-Controlled, Parallel-Group Study of the Efficacy, Safety, and Tolerability of THC:CBD Extract and	Peer-Reviewed, Clinical, Double-Blind	"The primary analysis of change from baseline in mean pain Numerical Rating Scale (NRS) score was statistically significantly in favor of THC: CBD compared with placebo... This study shows that THC: CBD extract is efficacious for relief of pain in patients with advanced cancer pain not fully relieved by

THC Extract in Patients with Intractable Cancer-Related Pain		strong opioids."
Cannabinoids: Potential Anticancer Agents	Peer-Reviewed, Literature Review	"Cannabinoids -- the active components of Cannabis sativa and their derivatives -- exert palliative effects in cancer patients by preventing nausea, vomiting and pain and by stimulating appetite. In addition, these compounds have been shown to inhibit the growth of tumor cells in culture and animal models by modulating key cell-signaling pathways. Cannabinoids are usually well tolerated, and do not produce the generalized toxic effects of conventional chemotherapies."
Marijuana as Antiemetic Medicine: A Survey of Oncologists' Experiences and Attitudes	Peer-Reviewed, Random Survey	"More than 44% of the respondents report recommending the (illegal) use of marijuana for the control of emesis to at least one cancer chemotherapy patient. Almost

one half (48%) would prescribe marijuana to some of their patients if it were legal. As a group, respondents considered smoked marijuana to be somewhat more effective than the legally available oral synthetic dronabinol ([THC] Marinol; Unimed, Somerville, NJ) and roughly as safe. Of the respondents who expressed an opinion, a majority (54%) thought marijuana should be available by prescription.

These results bear on the question of whether marijuana has a 'currently accepted medical use,' at issue in an ongoing administrative and legal dispute concerning whether marijuana in smoked form should be available by prescription along with synthetic THC in oral form. This survey demonstrates that oncologists' experience with the medical use of marijuana is more extensive, and their opinions of it are more favorable, than the regulatory

		authorities appear to have believed."
Marijuana: An Effective Antiepileptic Treatment in Partial Epilepsy? A Case Report and Review of the Literature	Peer-reviewed, Case Study, Literature Review	"Although more data are needed, animal studies and clinical experience suggest that marijuana or its active constituents may have a place in the treatment of partial epilepsy. [In the study] we present the case of a 45-year-old man with cerebral palsy and epilepsy who showed marked improvement with the use of marijuana. This case supports other anecdotal data suggesting that marijuana use may be a beneficial adjunctive treatment in some patients with epilepsy."
Marijuana Use and Epilepsy; Prevalence in Patients of a Tertiary Care Epilepsy Center	Peer-Reviewed, Survey	"Twenty-one percent of subjects had used marijuana in the past year with the majority of active users reporting beneficial effects on seizures. Twenty-four percent of all subjects believed marijuana was an effective therapy for epilepsy. Despite limited evidence of

| | | efficacy, many patients with epilepsy believe marijuana is an effective therapy for epilepsy and are actively using it." |

*gathered from procon.org, full references provided in References section

Chapter Four: Present Day Opinion in the United States

Opinions on the use of medical marijuana are changing in the United States, from the American Academy of Pediatrics, to the American Cancer Society to well-known physicians. Additionally, some figures in government and mainstream culture is beginning to reevaluate the use of marijuana for medical purposes (some citing more need for regulation than others), particularly when conditions for patients are "life-limiting or severely debilitating" (American Academy of Pediatrics, p.3, 2015). When examining the opinion of the medical field, the designation between recreational use and medical use becomes clearer, yet much of the federal government's stance is heavily based on fear and policy decisions and fails to access available scientific data. Furthermore, much of the government's stance fails to acknowledge current access to marijuana, recreationally, even amongst strict regulations. With election year nearing, however, medical marijuana is expected to take a front seat in the platform of candidates, including Hillary Clinton.

While the U.S. Federal Government's stance against medical marijuana includes concerns about increased access and inability to control the compound, even under strict control federally, marijuana is one of the leading substances accessed by people young and old in the United States recreationally. Additionally, some of the compounds used for treatment in medical marijuana do not provide the "high" typically associated with recreational use of marijuana, yet typically arguments against medical marijuana cite this property. While the pharmaceutical industry has created medical marijuana replacements such as Marinol, when the major and minor compounds of marijuana are separated, often the treatment for a host of symptoms is not as effective for some patients, yet work for others (United Patients Group, 2015). Differing results, restrictions by the federal government, decades-old stereotypical views of marijuana and confusion over medical versus recreational use create tension around the scientific plausibility that medical marijuana holds valuable information for a variety of diseases. Fortunately, in the medical community, the landscape is changing.

In a recent publication of WebMD, Rappold (2014) reported that a "majority of doctors say that medical marijuana should be legalized nationally and that it can deliver real benefits to patients." WebMD surveyed 1,544 doctors as a part of efforts to inform the public as more than 10 states were considering bills to legalize medical marijuana. In the survey, solid support for legalization efforts was found, with most doctors saying medical marijuana should be legal in their states and that medical marijuana should be an option for patients. WebMD's survey included doctors from more than 12 specialties and 48 states. From nationally recognized organizations, to well-known physicians, the changing landscape of the medical community's belief around medical marijuana is evident, in state legislation, in policy briefs and in practices around the country to treat disease.

Earlier this year, the Brookings Institute quoted an interview with CNN last year, in which Hillary Clinton signaled support for medical marijuana, research on the topic, and the rights of states to legalize recreational marijuana. Clinton stated, "...I think we need to be very clear about the benefits of marijuana use for medicinal purposes. I don't think we've done enough research yet, although I think for people who are in extreme medical conditions and have anecdotal evidence that it works, there should be availability under appropriate circumstances.... On recreational, you know, states are the laboratories of democracy. We have at least two states that are experimenting with that right now. I want to wait and see what the evidence is" (Brookings Institute, 2015).

In fact, medical marijuana and decriminalization of recreational marijuana are predicted to be an issue for presidential contenders in the 2016 election. While more and more states vote to approve decriminalizing marijuana use, Congress may be forced to reconsider rescheduling the substance. With increasing pressure from the public, regulations around medical marijuana and perhaps recreational use of marijuana as well, may look totally different in less than a decade. According to a 2014 Gallup Survey, 51 percent of Americans said they favor legalization of marijuana, according to the most recent Gallup survey. A decade ago, in 2004, nearly two-thirds of Americans were against legalization, marking an overall change in public perception.

In an article just published in National Geographic (June, 2015), the change from medicine to the illegal substance is described well, for most of the United States history, cannabis was legal:

"Then came Reefer Madness. Marijuana, the Assassin of Youth. The Killer Weed. The Gateway Drug. For nearly 70 years the plant went into hiding, and medical research largely stopped. In 1970 the federal government made it even harder to study marijuana, classifying it as a Schedule I drug—a dangerous substance with no valid medical purpose and a high potential for abuse, in the same category as heroin. In America most people expanding knowledge about cannabis were by definition criminals."

Of particular interest in the recent National Geographic article, is a visit Hampton Sides, author of the article, makes to Madrid to visit Manuel Guzmán. Guzmán is a biochemist and has studied cannabis for twenty years. While Guzmán is quick to point out "There are many claims on the Internet, but they are very, very weak," he is also eager to share his work. As described by Sides:

He [Guzmán] blinks thoughtfully, and then turns to his computer. "However, let me show you something." On his screen flash two MRIs of a rat's brain. The animal has a large mass lodged in the right hemisphere, caused by human brain tumor cells Guzmán's researchers injected. He zooms in. The mass bulges hideously. The rat, I think, is a goner. "This particular animal was treated with THC for one week," Guzmán continues. "And this is what happened afterward." The two images that now fill his screen are normal. The mass has not only shrunk—it's disappeared. "As you can see no tumor at all."

Guzmán's work, which has involved treating animals with cancer using cannabis for 15 years, has found that tumors were eradicated or reduced in two-thirds of those affected. According to Guzman, however, before people get too excited, they must consider "mice are not humans. We do not know if this can be extrapolated to humans at all."

Another interesting interview contained in the recent National Geographic article, introduces readers to the work of Nolan Kane. According to Kane, who has spent years working to secure permission and space to study the plant at the University of Colorado Boulder, "So much of science is incremental," …."but with this cannabis work, the science will not be incremental. It will be transformative. Transformative not just in our understanding of the plant but also of ourselves—our brains, our neurology, our psychology." Kane continues on, describing his current work and desire to assemble a map of the cannabis genome. Kane believes this will be "transformative in terms of the biochemistry of its compounds. Transformative in terms of its impact across several different industries, including medicine, agriculture, and biofuels. It may even transform part of our diet—hemp seed is known to be a ready source of very healthy, protein-rich oil" (Sides, 2015).

Chapter Five: Four Case Studies from American Survivors

Charlotte Figi's Story

Charlotte Figi is now eight years old, at the time her and her family's story went live on CNN, she was six. At the time her parents, Matt and Paige Figi decided to try medical marijuana as a last resort, Charlotte was five years old and was suffering from "300 grand mal seizures a week" and was in hospice preparing for an order her parents placed, "do not resuscitate" (Young, 2013). Charlotte had her first seizure in 2006, when she was 3 months old.

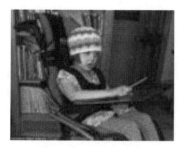

After conducting every test, no cause could be found and as Charlotte grew, the seizures continued. Matt and Paige continued to provide Charlotte with medications recommended by pediatricians, yet she stopped developing cognitively. Eventually Charlotte was diagnosed with a severe form of epilepsy, Dravet Syndrome. After doing some research, Matt Figi discovered the case of a boy with Dravet who'd been helped by low-level THC medical marijuana. In a recent article posted by Figi on www.theroc.us, Charlotte stated

"My six year old daughter, Charlotte, is diagnosed with Dravet Syndrome; a catastrophic pediatric epilepsy. She has significant cognitive and motor delays, brain damage, a surgically placed feeding tube for water and food, struggles to talk and walk, and needs full care in all areas of life...

After getting the green light from our team of neurologists and pediatricians, we started Charlotte at low, non-psychoactive doses [of cannabis] and charted her progress. The first week she went seven days seizure-free, down from the 300 grand mals she had the previous week. Three months into our journey and she was at a solid 90% seizure reduction and free of all pharmaceuticals. Eight months into our journey put her at 99+% seizure reduction.

Along with the seizure control, there are many other benefits she is experiencing from the medical cannabis. Despite being previously 100% tube-fed, she is consistently eating and drinking on her own for the first time in years. She sleeps soundly through the night. Her severe autism-like behaviors of self-injury, stimming, crying, violence, no eye contact, zero sleep, lack of social contact... are a thing of the past. She is clear-headed, focused, and has no attention deficit. Charlotte rides horses, skis, paints, dances, hikes. She even has friends for the first time. Her brain is healing. She is healthy. She is happy."

www.facebook.com/officialbookpageforcuringcancer

www.crushitwithkdp.com

Rick Simpson's Story

Rick Simpson's journey started in 2003. In 2003, Simpson was diagnosed with skin cancer. The cancerous spots were found on his face and neck. Simpson tried surgery on one of the spots, but saw little success. Simpson had been using cannabis oil for other health reasons due to an accident at the hospital he had worked at for 25 years. In 1997, while working on some pipes at the hospital, Simpson sustained a head injury. After the head injury, Simpson suffered a severe post-concussion syndrome and was prescribed pharmaceuticals, which led to severe side effects, including leaving him unable to function in day to day life.

After failed attempts at recovery from the hospital accident, Simpson was tipped off about medical marijuana by a television show, *The Nature of Things* and began smoking marijuana daily. He had saw improvement in pain, sensory disorder (hearing) and an improvement in his blood pressure from using marijuana following his hospital injury. After some time, both the post-concussion syndrome and effects of the pharmaceuticals were greatly reduced. Because Simpson's doctor discouraged him from smoking marijuana, he began experimenting with creating cannabis oil, by extracting the oil from whole plants (Coldwell, 2014).

When many years later his doctor suggested surgery for the skin cancer on his face, he recalled the radio headline had stated that the "University of Virginia had found the cannabinoid in cannabis THC could kill cancer in mice." Based off his results in treating himself following his hospital accident and the radio headline he heard some thirty years prior, he figured "that if it kills cancer in mice it would kill his cancer too" (http://www.cureyourowncancer.org, accessed May, 2015). According to Simpson's website (phoenixtears.ca), after four days of leaving cannabis oil on the cancerous spots on his neck and face, the cancer was gone. Unlike the surgery on one of the spots, the cannabis oil appeared to be effective.

Dennis Hill's Story

Dennis Hill is a biochemist who claims to have cured his Stage 4 prostate cancer. Hill attended post-graduate studies at Baylor Medical School, and later worked in cancer research at M.D. Anderson hospital for ten years, and in hospital administration for another ten years after completing his M.B.A. studies at St. Edwards University, Houston. In 1993, Hill transitioned to work in software engineering. Currently Hill is working on software projects and teaching meditation and was recently brought on to Stevia's advisory panel. In 2010 after a regularly scheduled visit to his physician, Hill was diagnosed "with very aggressive adenocarcinoma in his prostate gland." Adenocarcinoma attacks the body by targeting mucus secreting glands throughout the body (Real Hemp, 2015). Early prostate cancer usually causes no symptoms, which is why early detection testing is recommended for men beginning at age 50. According to the American Cancer Society (2015) advanced prostate cancers can include symptoms, such as:

- Problems urinating, including a slow or weak urinary stream or the need to urinate more often, especially at night.
- Blood in the urine
- Trouble getting an erection (erectile dysfunction)
- Pain in the hips, back (spine), chest (ribs), or other areas from cancer spread to bones

- Weakness or numbness in the legs or feet, or even loss of bladder or bowel control from cancer pressing on the spinal cord.

In a statement by Dennis Hill, posted on a popular pro-medical marijuana website https://patients4medicalmarijuana.wordpress.com (May 15, 2015), Hill shared the following in 2013:

"Three years ago, after a prostate biopsy, I was given the diagnosis of aggressive Stage III adenocarcinoma. I didn't know what to do. The urologist made appointments for me to start radiation, and maybe chemo. Then a friend told me *cannabis cures cancer*. It just so happened that the first human trials of cannabis treatment of astrocytomas (inoperable brain cancer), were published with encouraging results. So I decided; rather than die from the medical treatment, I would do the cannabis cure. Now... where to get some. There was no dispensary in the area, but a friend made me cannabis butter, so I took that, up to tolerance. In three months the primary cancer was gone, only minor metastatic lesions were left. At that point I found a supplier for Rick Simpson oil and killed off the metastases in the next three months. Now I just take a maintenance dose of locally produced hash oil that is 1:1 THC: CBD with about a 30% potency. This will certainly keep me clear of cancer, anywhere, forever. My point in telling this story is the fact that in the face of advanced aggressive cancer, all I had was very weak cannabutter, but it was enough to eliminate the primary tumor. Now there are strains of 95% THC. But is this necessary? If you have cancer and want to pursue the cannabis treatment, any at all will be good. More important than extreme potency, is balance between THC and CBD. If you can get high potency, great. If not, common potencies will work perfectly. Finally, if you choose cannabinoid treatment, start small, then increase dosage as rapidly as tolerable. To kill cancer you have to hit it hard, be conscientious about your treatment. Cannabis does no harm to the body; it is a metabolic support for the immune system. Here are the basics, based on my own experience with cancer and cannabis oil extract.

- Get Rick Simpson formula oil; including the important decarboxylation step to convert THCA to THC.
- If possible, use 1:1 THC: CBD, as THC kills the cancer, CBD kills the cancer's ability to metastasize.
- Take as much as possible; the way to kill cancer is to hit it very hard. Start very small to acclimate to the oil properties, and then keep increasing the dose as tolerable.
- Take a large dose before bed, then a lighter dose during the day, to keep the pressure on the cancer."

Ed Moore's Story

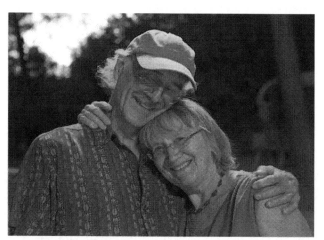

Photo credit: chrisbeatcancer.com

Ed Moore, pictured with his wife of over 35 years above, is a survivor of Stage 4 liver cancer. After visiting the local hospital and realizing cancer had spread to cover part of his lower lobe and had blocked his bile duct, he went home with his wife in 2012, expecting no recovery. In a statement posted on the Facebook page "Cannabis Cures Cancer" Moore states the following:

> "I'm Ed and we're going to tell you a little bit about my cancer survival. ...
>
> In April of ... 2012, I was diagnosed with 4th stage liver cancer...
>
> The hospital said it was inoperable, it was too far advanced ... that basically they were going to hook me up with hospice and send me home to stay comfortable

until I died, which they said would be within 2 weeks to 2 months, a couple of the doctors said 2, 3 months.

And I lost a lot of weight, started turning grey, my bones stuck out ... my friends would come to see me and start crying because they thought I was going to die any minute, or the next day or two ... and I kind of thought I was too, I thought I was really sick.

After leaving the hospital after a short stay, Moore left to return home and was given morphine to help with the pain. According to Moore's wife, the morphine made him vomit and affected his mind. After choosing a Naturopath doctor, the Moore's began using their own cannabis to produce Phoenix Tears, the cannabis oil based off Rick Simpson's formula. Within one week, Moore reports he "was off the morphine." In addition to consuming the cannabis oil, Moore began juicing fresh buds and leaves mixed with vegetables. Within two weeks, Moore reports "his pain and swollen stomach disappeared." In addition to cannabis oil, Moore began taking Vitamin C, intravenously and spends time daily using a sauna, Epsom salt bath and castor oil packs to rid his body of toxins. While not completely "in the clear" according to the Moore's self-maintained website http://cannabis-cancer-info.org, Moore has had "three years of quality life" as of April, 2015. Moore continues a strict protocol for health, which can be accessed on his website and continues using cannabis oil.

www.facebook.com/officialbookpageforcuringcancer

Appendix: Government Contacts

Resources:

    Interested in impacting regulations on medical marijuana in your home state? Reach out to your senator!

    The United States Congress has an upper chamber called the Senate and a lower chamber called the House of Representatives (or "House" for short) which share the responsibilities of the legislative process to create federal statutory law. Listings by state were retrieved from www.govtrack.us and each Senator's home state website was visited to verify and research contact information (May, 2015).

www.facebook.com/officialbookpageforcuringcancer

Senator	State	Contact Information
RICHARD SHELBY	Alabama	304 Russell Senate Office Building Washington, DC 20510 (202) 224-5744
JEFFERSON "JEFF" SESSIONS	Alabama	326 Russell Senate Office Building Washington, DC 20510 (202) 224-4124
LISA MURKOWSKI	Alaska	709 Hart Senate Building Washington, D.C. 20510 (202) 224-6665
DAN SULLIVAN	Alaska	B40A Dirksen Senate Office Building Washington, DC 20510 (202) 224-3004
JOHN MCCAIN	Arizona	241 Russell Senate Office Building Washington, DC 20510

www.crushitwithkdp.com

www.facebook.com/officialbookpageforcuringcancer

			(202) 224-2235
JEFF FLAKE	Arizona		Senate Russell Office Building 413 Washington, D.C. 20510 (202) 224-4521
JOHN BOOZMAN	Arkansas		141 Hart Senate Office Building Washington, DC 20510 (202) 224-4843
Tom Cotton	Arkansas		B-33 Russell Senate Office Building Washington, DC 20510 (202) 224-2353
DIANNE FEINSTEIN	California		United States Senate 331 Hart Senate Office Building Washington, D.C. 20510 (202) 224-3841
BARBARA BOXER	California		112 Hart Senate Office Building Washington, D.C. 20510 (202) 224-3553

www.crushitwithkdp.com

www.facebook.com/officialbookpageforcuringcancer

MICHAEL BENNET	Colorado	261 Russell Senate Office Building Washington, DC 20510 (202) 224-5852
Cory Gardner	Colorado	Senate Dirksen Office Building SD-B40B Washington, DC 20510 (202) 224-5941
RICHARD BLUMENTHAL	Connecticut	706 Hart Senate Office Bldg. Washington, DC, 20510 (202) 224-2823
CHRISTOPHER MURPHY	Connecticut	136 Hart Senate Office Bldg. Washington, DC 20510 (202) 224-4041
THOMAS CARPER	Delaware	513 Hart Senate Office Building Washington, DC 20510 (202) 224-2441

www.crushitwithkdp.com

www.facebook.com/officialbookpageforcuringcancer

CHRIS COONS	Delaware	127A Russell Senate Office Building Washington, D.C. 20510 (202) 224-5042
Bill Nelson	Florida	716 Hart Senate Office Building Washington DC 20510 (202) 224-5274
Marco Rubio	Florida	284 Russell Senate Office Building Washington DC 20510 (202) 224-3041
Johnny Isakson	Georgia	131 Russell Senate Office Building Washington DC 20510 (202) 224-3643
David Perdue	Georgia	B40D Dirksen Senate Office Building Washington DC 20510 202) 224-3521

www.crushitwithkdp.com

Mazie Hirono	Hawaii	330 Hart Senate Office Building Washington DC 20510 202) 224-6361
Mike Crapo	Idaho	239 Dirksen Senate Office Building Washington, D.C. 20510 (202) 224-6142
RICHARD DURBIN	Illinois	711 Hart Senate Building Washington, D.C. 20510 (202) 224.2152
MARK KIRK	Illinois	524 Hart Senate Office Building Washington DC, 20510 (202) 224-2854
DANIEL COATS	Indiana	493 Russell Office Bldg. Washington, D.C. 20510 (202) 224-5623

JOE DONNELLY	Indiana	720 Hart Senate Office Building Washington, D.C. 20510 (202) 224-4814
CHARLES "CHUCK" GRASSLEY	Iowa	135 Hart Senate Office Building Washington, D.C. 20510 (202) 224-3744
JONI ERNST	Iowa	825 B/C Hart Senate Office Building Washington, DC 20510 (202) 224-3254
PAT ROBERTS	Kansas	109 Hart Senate Office Building Washington, DC 20510-1605 (202) 224-4774
JERRY MORAN	Kansas	Dirksen Senate Office Building Room 521 Washington, D.C. 20510 (202) 224-6521

MITCH MCCONNELL	Kentucky	317 Russell Senate Office Building Washington, DC 20510 (202) 224-2541
RAND PAUL	Kentucky	167 Russell Senate Office Building Washington DC, 20510 (202) 224-4343
DAVID VITTER	Louisiana	516 Hart Senate Office Building Washington, DC 20510 (202) 224-4623
BILL CASSIDY	Louisiana	703 Hart Senate Office Building Washington, DC 20510 (202) 224-5824
SUSAN COLLINS	Maine	413 Dirksen Senate Office Building Washington, DC 20510 (202) 224-2523

ANGUS KING	Maine	133 Hart Building Washington, D.C. 20510 (202) 224-5344
BARBARA MIKULSKI	Maryland	503 Hart Senate Office Building Washington, D.C., 20510 (202) 224-4654
BENJAMIN CARDIN	Maryland	509 Hart Senate Office Building Washington, DC, 20510 (202) 224-4524
ELIZABETH WARREN	Massachusetts	317 Hart Senate Office Building Washington, DC 20510 (202) 224-4543
EDWARD "ED" MARKEY	Massachusetts	255 Dirksen Senate Office Building Washington, D.C. 20510 (202) 224-2742

www.facebook.com/officialbookpageforcuringcancer

DEBBIE STABENOW	Michigan	731 Hart Senate Office Building Washington, DC 20510 (202) 224-4822
GARY PETERS	Michigan	SRC-2 Russell Senate Office Building Washington, DC 20510 (202) 224-6221
AMY KLOBUCHAR	Minnesota	302 Hart Senate Office Building Washington, DC 20510 (202) 224-3244
ALAN "AL" FRANKEN	Minnesota	309 Hart Senate Office Building Washington, DC 20510 (202) 224-5641
THAD COCHRAN	Mississippi	113 Dirksen Senate Office Building Washington, D.C. 20510 (202) 224-5054
ROGER WICKER	Mississippi	555 Dirksen Senate Office Building

www.crushitwithkdp.com

www.facebook.com/officialbookpageforcuringcancer

		Washington, DC 20510 (202) 224-6253
CLAIRE MCCASKILL	Missouri	730 Hart Senate Office Building Washington, D.C. 20510 (202) 224-6154
ROY BLUNT	Missouri	260 Russell Senate Office Building Washington, DC 20510 (202) 224-5721
JON TESTER	Montana	311 Hart Senate Office Building Washington, DC 20510-2604 (202) 224-2644
STEVE DAINES	Montana	320 Hart Senate Office Building Washington, DC 20510 (202) 224-2651
DEB FISCHER	Nebraska	454 Russell Senate Office Building Washington, DC 20510 (202) 224-6551

www.crushitwithkdp.com

BENJAMIN SASSE	Nebraska	B40E Dirksen Senate Office Building Washington, DC 20510 (202) 224-4224
HARRY REID	Nevada	522 Hart Senate Office Building Washington, DC 20510 (202) 224-3542
DEAN HELLER	Nevada	324 Hart Senate Office Building Washington, DC 20510 (202) 224-6244
JEANNE SHAHEEN	New Hampshire	506 Hart Senate Office Building Washington, DC 20510 (202) 224-2841
KELLY AYOTTE	New Hampshire	144 Russell Senate Office Building Washington, D.C. 20510 (202) 224-3324
ROBERT "BOB"	New Jersey	528 Senate Hart Office Building

www.facebook.com/officialbookpageforcuringcancer

MENÉNDEZ		Washington, D.C. 20510 (202) 224-4744
CORY BOOKER	New Jersey	359 Dirksen Senate Office Building Washington, DC 20510 (202) 224-3224
TOM UDALL	New Mexico	531 Hart Senate Office Building Washington DC, 20510 (202) 224-6621
MARTIN HEINRICH	New Mexico	303 Hart Senate Office Building Washington, D.C. 20510 (202) 224-5521
CHARLES "CHUCK" SCHUMER	New York	322 Hart Senate Office Building Washington, D.C. 20510 (202) 224-6542
KIRSTEN GILLIBRAND	New York	478 Russell Washington, DC 20510 (202) 224-4451
RICHARD BURR	North Carolina	217 Russell Senate Office

www.crushitwithkdp.com

		Building Washington, DC 20510 (202) 224-3154
THOM TILLIS	North Carolina	G55 Dirksen Senate Office Building Washington, DC 20510 (202) 224-6342
JOHN HOEVEN	North Dakota	338 Russell Senate Office Bldg. Washington DC, 20510 (202) 224-2551
HEIDI HEITKAMP	North Dakota	SH-110 Hart Senate Office Building Washington, DC 20510 (202) 224-2043
SHERROD BROWN	Ohio	713 Hart Senate Office Bldg. Washington, DC 20510 tel: (202) 224-2315

www.facebook.com/officialbookpageforcuringcancer

ROBERT "ROB" PORTMAN	Ohio	448 Russell Senate Office Building Washington, DC 20510 (202) 224-3353
JAMES "JIM" INHOFE	Oklahoma	205 Russell Senate Office Building Washington, DC 20510 (202) 224-4721
JAMES LANKFORD	Oklahoma	316 Hart Senate Office Building Washington, DC 20510 (202) 224-5754
RON WYDEN	Oregon	221 Dirksen Senate Office Bldg. Washington, D.C., 20510 (202) 224-5244
JEFF MERKLEY	Oregon	313 Hart Senate Office Building Washington, DC 20510 (202) 224-3753
ROBERT "BOB"	Pennsylvania	393 Russell Senate Office

CASEY JR.		Building Washington, D.C. 20510 (202) 224-6324
PATRICK "PAT" TOOMEY	Pennsylvania	248 Russell Senate Office Building Washington, D.C. 20510 (202) 224-4254
JOHN "JACK" REED	Rhode Island	728 Hart Senate Office Building Washington, DC 20510 (202) 224-4642
SHELDON WHITEHOUSE	Rhode Island	Hart Senate Office Bldg. Room 530 Washington, DC, 20510 (202) 224-2921
LINDSEY GRAHAM	South Carolina	290 Russell Senate Office Building Washington, DC 20510 (202) 224-5972
TIM SCOTT	South Carolina	520 Hart Senate Office Building

www.facebook.com/officialbookpageforcuringcancer

		Washington, DC 20510 (202) 224-6121

www.crushitwithkdp.com

JOHN THUNE	South Dakota	United States Senate SD-511 Washington, DC 20510 (202) 224-2321
MIKE ROUNDS	South Dakota	Russell Senate Office Building Courtyard 4 Washington, DC 20510 (202) 224-5842
LAMAR ALEXANDER	Tennessee	455 Dirksen Senate Office Building Washington, DC 20510 (202) 224-4944
BOB CORKER	Tennessee	Dirksen Senate Office Building SD-425 Washington, DC 20510 (202) 224-3344
JOHN CORNYN	Texas	517 Hart Senate Office Bldg. Washington, DC 20510 (202) 224-2934
TED CRUZ	Texas	404 Russell Washington, DC 20510

www.facebook.com/officialbookpageforcuringcancer

			(202) 224-5922
ORRIN HATCH	Utah		104 Hart Office Washington, DC 20510
MIKE LEE	Utah		361A Russell Senate Office Building Washington, D.C. 20510 (202) 224-5444
PATRICK LEAHY	Vermont		437 Russell Senate Bldg. United States Senate Washington, DC 20510 (202) 224-4242
BERNARD "BERNIE" SANDERS	Vermont		332 Dirksen Building Washington, D.C. 20510 tel: (202) 224-5141
MARK WARNER	Virginia		475 Russell Senate Office Building Washington, DC 20510 202-224-2023

www.crushitwithkdp.com

TIMOTHY KAINE	Virginia	388 Russell Senate Office Building Washington, D.C. 20510 (202) 224-4024
PATTY MURRAY	Washington	154 Russell Senate Office Building Washington, D.C. 20510 (202) 224-2621
MARIA CANTWELL	Washington	511 Hart Senate Office Building Washington, D.C. 20510 (202) 224-3441
JOE MANCHIN III	West Virginia	306 Hart Senate Office Building Washington DC, 20510 202-224-3954
SHELLEY CAPITO	West Virginia	172 Russell Senate Office Building Washington, DC 20510 (202) 224-6472

RON JOHNSON	Wisconsin	328 Hart Senate Office Building Washington, DC 20510 (202) 224-5323
TAMMY BALDWIN	Wisconsin	717 Hart Senate Office Building Washington, D.C. 20510 (202) 224-565
JOHN BARRASSO	Wyoming	307 Dirksen Senate Office Building Washington, DC 20510 (202) 224-6441
Michael Enzi	Wyoming	379A Senate Russell Office Building Washington, DC 20510 (202) 224-3424

References:

Brookings Institute, (2015, May). 12 People to Watch: http://www.brookings.edu/blogs/fixgov/posts/2015/04/20-420-series-12-people-to-watch-hudak

Coldwell, L. (2014). Rick Simpson's Canadian Cancer Cures and the Rising Cannabis Oil Movement. Retrieved May 18, 2015, from http://drleonardcoldwell.com

Genetic Science Learning Center (2014, June 22) Cannabis in the Clinic: The Medical Marijuana Debate, *Learn Genetics*. Retrieved May 06, 2015, from http://learn.genetics.utah.edu/content/addiction/cannabis/

Grinspoon, L. (2007). Boston Globe, 2007. "Marijuana as a Wonder Drug"
http://medicalmarijuana.procon.org/view.answers.php?questionID=000087&print=true

Gupta, Sanjay (August 5, 2013), *"Weed: Dr. Sanjay Gupta Reports" premieres Sunday, 8/11 8p ET*, CNN, retrieved January 1, 2014

New York Times (2015, May) Marijuana Topics. http://topics.nytimes.com/top/reference/timestopics/subjects/m/marijuana/index.html
Pediatrics; originally published online January 26, 2015; DOI: 10.1542/peds.2014-4146. The Impact of

www.facebook.com/officialbookpageforcuringcancer

Marijuana Policies on Youth: Clinical, Research, and Legal Update.

Sides, H. (2015). *Science Seeks to Unlock Marijuana's Secrets.* National Geographic, retrieved May 18, 2015.

Young, Saundra (August 7, 2013), *Marijuana stops child's severe seizures*, CNN, retrieved January 1, 2014

Walia, Arjun (2014, May). A Recipe to make Cannabis Oil. http://www.collective-evolution.com/2014/06/29/a-recipe-to-make-cannabis-oil-for-a-chemotherapy-alternative/

White House (2015, May). Marijuana Info. http://www.whitehouse.gov/marijuanainfo

THE END OR MAYBE IT'S THE BEGINNING!!!

KING CAJUN

KingCajun Publishing

YALL COME SEE US, YA HEAR!!!

GET YOUR COPY OF PALEO GRUBS TODAY!
http://bit.ly/kingcajun

3 WEEK DIET SYSTEM - 12 TO 23 POUNDS IN 21 DAYS! LOSE 2 TO 3 INCHES!
We believe you will benefit from this program so check it out now!

www.crushitwithkdp.com

www.facebook.com/officialbookpageforcuringcancer

www.crushitwithkdp.com

Made in the USA
Middletown, DE
06 November 2019